1

Thyroid Hormones and the Tests That Monitor Them

Hormonal Functions, Imbalances and Treatments

By: James M. Lowrance © 2008

ABOUT THE AUTHOR:

I am a husband, father, grandfather and lifetime contract salesman, with experience in health writing that began in 2004. I completed theological studies with Liberty University in 1996. I formerly served as editor and forum moderator of Thyroid Health for BellaOnline.com and as a general health writer for Suite101.com, where I received Editor's Choice Awards for my articles on health subjects.

In 2003 I was diagnosed with hypothyroidism; "Hashimoto's thyroiditis" being the cause. This autoimmune form of thyroid disease that causes destruction of the thyroid gland resulted in my also developing "Chronic Fatigue Syndrome", due to a compromised immune system with severe co-morbid "Adrenal Fatigue". I also suffered severe anxiety symptoms, including panic attacks early into the onset of Hashimoto's thyroiditis (Hashitoxicosis). A common heart murmur I was diagnosed with in my teens called "Mitral Valve Prolapse", also worsened in severity of symptoms, with the development of these other health disorders.

My eventual receiving of diagnoses was a difficult process with proper diagnostic testing not being ordered by the first doctors I sought treatment from. These types of issues were inspiration for me to become proactive in my own health care and to self-educate myself on these health disorders, which I have done extensively since 2003. I now enjoy sharing this information with other patients experiencing my same health disorders.

TABLE OF CONTENTS:

<u>Chapter One</u>

The Purpose of Thyroid Function Hormones

There are four major hormones having to do with thyroid function and the resulting metabolism these regulate within the body. In this chapter we will look at the purposes of the thyroid related hormones called the T-4, T-3, Reverse T-3 and TSH. The chapters following will include a good deal of information covering the TSH hormone because of its prominence in diagnosing thyroid hormone imbalances, at their earliest stages and due to its use in monitoring treated hypothyroid patients, who are dosed with prescribed hormone therapies.

The thyroid is mostly comprised-of or made up of an element called "iodine". This iodine is produced and made available in the thyroid gland through cells called hormones, each containing a certain number of iodine molecules. These manufactured thyroid hormones are then sent from the thyroid gland, for disbursement throughout the body, in order to regulate the metabolism or the rate at which the body functions and burns energy.

The two major thyroid hormones "T-4" and "T-3" are sometimes blood tested together or separately to detect abnormally low or abnormally high levels of them, caused by thyroid hormone imbalances (disorders).

Thyroxine (T-4)

The most abundant thyroid hormone in the body is the one called "thyroxine" (T-4). This is the hormone produced in larger amounts by the thyroid gland, so that there is an adequate supply of it to be converted into a more active form of thyroid hormone (T-3) which is more responsible for regulating the metabolism of the body. T-4 itself, in its pre-conversion form, is less metabolically active than is T-3. Thyroxine contains four molecules of iodine, which is why it is commonly abbreviated as "T-4". You could say that the T-4 hormone is a reserve/precursor hormone that is ready to be converted into the more metabolically active T-3 hormone.

Despite the fact that T-4 contains one more iodine molecule, the T-3 hormone (described in more detail below) is at least five times more powerful than T-4.

The T-4 hormone is the less metabolically inactive of the two as previously stated and it is stored in the body until converted into T-3, as the body needs it. This conversion process is accomplished via enzymes or proteins found within the body thatattach to the T-4 hormone cells, turning them into T-3, as the body needs an increase in the rate of metabolism. The need for metabolism increases can be due to changes in physical activity and to utilize energy from things that are consumed, including food, water and oxygen intake. The two major protein/enzymes that are involved in this process, are the "thyroid peroxidase" and the "thyroglobulin". The conversion process is believed to take place mainly within the liver and partially within the kidneys as well.

Triiodothyronine (T-3)

The second major thyroid hormone, and the one that has been described as being more powerful in regard to regulating bodily metabolism, is medically referred to as "triiodothyronine" (T-3). This is the thyroid hormone converted from T-4 as described previously.

This one contains only three molecules of iodine, but is many times more powerful than the T-4 hormone (some medical sources state that T-3 is estimated to be from 5 to 10 times more powerful than T-4). The conversion process from T-4 to T-3 is accomplished through the enzyme/proteins, listed in the previous subheading, that enter into the T-4 hormone cells and cause them to convert into T-3 hormone cells as needed. With this process taking place mainly within the liver, this demonstrates one of the many important purposes of the liver in helping to regulate bodily metabolism, via cooperation with the endocrine system (i.e. the pituitary, thyroid and adrenal glands).

Reverse R-3 (R T-3)

When the body has converted enough T-3 from the T-4 hormone, it will then convert any of the excess T-4 hormones into another type of inactive hormone called "Reverse T-3" (R T-3). This is another function that takes place within the liver, to eliminate any extra T-4 produced by the thyroid gland.

The conversion of the extra hormone into Reverse T-3 protects the body against having too much of the powerful T-3 hormone, which could stimulate an overactive metabolism should it reach abnormally high levels (hyperthyroidism).

This is how the body rids itself of extra T-4 in the body that is in excess to the amount needed to be stored and converted into T-3. Reverse T-3 is a term that actually means that the excess T-4 hormone has been rendered inactive (reversal of its metabolic action), so that too much of it is not converted into T-3, causing hyperthyroid states or what is also referred to as an overactive thyroid gland.

Certain diseases in the body and periods of extreme prolonged stress can cause the body to convert too much of the T-4 hormone into Reverse T-3, rather than into T-3, which is sometimes referred to as "euthroid sick syndrome". This will cause a slowed-down metabolism from lack of active thyroid hormone, which results in a type of "hypothyroidism" that is usually intermittent and temporary.

Problems with imbalances of Reverse T-3 are less common causes of hypothyroidism than are diseases directly affecting the thyroid gland or what is medically referred to as "primary hypothyroidism" and they are also rare compared to the types caused by a dysfunction of the master brain glands that help regulate thyroid function (i.e. the hypothalamus and pituitary), which is referred to as "Secondary" or "Central" Hypothyroidism. Some of the rare types of low thyroid hormone conditions are usually also temporary and can be corrected with short term T-3 hormone replacement therapy, as prescribed and administered by a qualified medical doctor. Others can be permanent (i.e. autoimmune types) and will require permanent/lifelong treatment.

Patients, who are treated for hypothyroidism, sometimes are found to have "impaired T-4 to T-3 conversion". These are patients who for some reason do not have the ability within their bodies, to adequately convert enough T-4 into the also needed T-3 hormone. Doctors do not always identify the problem that results in impaired conversion.

It may at times be due to an inability of the liver to aid in the conversion process, due to diseases affecting the organ (i.e. severe fatty liver disease or types of hepatitis).

There may also be co-morbid (co-existing) illness or disease of other kinds in the body that hinder the conversion process of T-4 to T-3 (i.e. heart or kidney disease). Regardless of the cause that may or may not be found (some cases are "idiopathic" -- meaning no cause is found) , these patients will need to have the low T-3 hormone replaced with thyroid hormone replacement therapy that includes both T-4 and T-3, rather than with a T-4 only thyroid hormone medication.

Unfortunately, some Doctors do not believe impaired conversion of T-4 to T-3 occurs, except in extremely rare cases and this will result in less blood testing of treated hypothyroid patients, of both their T-4 and T-3 levels because testing of these will be deemed unnecessary. These Doctors will believe the T-4 and T-3 tests are not necessary and they will only monitor treated hypothyroid patients with T-4 and TSH blood tests only.

The TSH or "Thyroid Stimulating Hormone" is not a thyroid hormone but is a pituitary hormone as discussed earlier that indicates/reflects how much thyroid hormone is available to the body in the blood stream. The problem however, with not testing both T-4 and T-3 levels in patients who are being treated for hypothyroidism with a T-4 only medication, at least for the first one or two follow up blood retests, is that adequate T-4 in the blood will give a normal TSH reading even when the T-3 hormone level may be clinically low.

The T-4 and T-3 blood tests come in a variety of different versions, such as the "totals" of each or the "free" levels of each (the latter being most recommended by thyroid specialists), or are combined in tests called the "FTI Index" and the "T-7".

There is also one called the "T-3 Uptake" that may be included in a thyroid panel but this one is usually only tested to diagnose thyroid disease but not as a follow-up on thyroid hormone replacement therapy (it doesn't measure T-3 levels but measures how much binding-globulin is available for the hormone to work properly in the body -- "uptake" capability).

Thyroid Hormones and the Tests That Monitor Them

All of these help determine thyroid hormone production levels and all of them have lab ranges with a "below-normal" indicating hypothyroidism and an "above-normal" indicating hyperthyroidism.

Thyroid Stimulating Hormone (TSH)

The hormone that regulates the rate at which the thyroid gland produces the T-4 hormone is called "Thyroid Stimulating Hormone" (TSH), which is sent from the pituitary gland in the brain-center. The production of T-4 will then result in the conversion of it into the needed T-3 (the more powerful metabolic hormone discussed previously) and Reverse T-3 (inactivated hormone). The TSH hormone comes from the pituitary, which continually monitors and communicates with the thyroid gland, in regard to how much T-4 hormone is in the blood and whether or not increases or decreases of it are needed at each given moment during life activities. If the pituitary gland detects that the thyroid gland is producing too much T-4 hormone, it will send less TSH to stimulate the thyroid gland to do so.

Thyroid Hormones and the Tests That Monitor Them

If the pituitary gland senses that the thyroid gland is not producing enough T-4 hormone it will send more TSH to stimulate it to do so. The TSH level when blood tested gives an accurate reflective-measure of how well the thyroid is functioning, in producing its own hormones.

Adversely, TSH is low when the thyroid is overactive and high when it is under-active, while the T-4 and T-3 will correlate as low with an under-active thyroid and high when the thyroid is overactive. Stated in simple terms, the thyroid hormone levels indicate the opposite to what the TSH level is indicating in regard to high and low levels that are occurring within the body, which can be changed overtly (significantly) when thyroid diseases of either the hypothyroid or hyperthyroid types are present. A healthy thyroid gland will have normal amounts of TSH stimulating it and when blood levels of TSH are tested in people suspected of having either an over-functioning or under-functioning thyroid gland, they can see from test results, if the pituitary gland is sending too much TSH (hypothyroidism) or too little TSH (hyperthyroidism) to stimulate production of T-4.

TSH tests will usually detect thyroid hormone imbalances earlier than any other blood test that is available and some doctors will choose to order it as a stand-alone test, before resorting to more extensive thyroid panels.

<u>Chapter Two</u>

The Best Blood Tests of Thyroid Function

In my opinion as a layperson and treated hypothyroid patient who has extensively researched this subject and corresponded with 1000s of patients since year-2003, treated hypothyroid patients need to have their "Free T-4" and "Free T-3" levels (the "frees" are the tests of unbound, available hormone) tested, in addition to TSH, for at least the first two blood retests, in follow up on their T-4 only thyroid hormone replacement therapy.

If these first follow up tests indicate that the hormone medication is resulting in adequate amounts of T-4 and T-3 (the latter being supplied through proper conversion), TSH only testing afterward, would be sufficient for follow up retests, to monitor the hormone replacement therapy.

The preceding paragraph was intended as a general description of thyroid hormones and the blood tests used to monitor them.

When thyroid hormone imbalances are detected however, other types of blood testing may be ordered to detect the "cause" of the thyroid hormone imbalance.

Tests for example, to detect "thyroid auto-antibodies" which are immune system cells that can mistakenly attack the thyroid gland and cause it to produce imbalanced amounts of hormones might be ordered as well.

If "thyroid autoimmunity", which is the most common cause of thyroid disorders in most industrialized countries, is not found, blood tests of pituitary function may also be ordered, to test for central (brain-center) causes of thyroid hormone imbalance.

In more complicated cases, hypothyroidism might be secondary to another disease process in the body, in which case, extensive blood testing of all types may then be undertaken to determine the cause of the thyroid hormone imbalance.

Thyroid Hormones and the Tests That Monitor Them

There are other diagnostic tests of thyroid function available, in addition to blood testing as well, such as radiological and ultrasound imaging tests and thyroid tissue biopsies. These will usually follow blood testing to detect thyroid hormone imbalances, when they are determined to be needed.

Chapter Three

Interpreting Your Blood Lab Results

In this chapter, I wish to discuss the importance of diagnostic blood testing and in that of patient-involvement in understanding their blood test results and in inquiring with their doctors as to which tests may be needed (patient proactive-ness can result in better treatment outcomes according to medical research studies).

Ask for copies of your blood lab reports (results).

If you have thyroid hormone blood tests done, request copies of the results from your doctor's office or from the blood laboratory that performed the tests. If you live in the USA, you are entitled to copies of results from blood tests that have been ordered for you. The law that obliges medical entities to provide copies to patients is called the "HIPAA Law." Once you have requested lab result copies of your personal tests, the office or lab has 30 days, according to this provision to comply with your request.

Once you receive copies, it is a good idea to make a notebook or file for your lab results that you can retain as back-up files, in the event you decide to see a new doctor (second opinion) or change doctors, without informing your previous doctor that you have decided to do so. Having your own copies is also helpful, in case you wish to post your results to a physician forum or patient forum online for further comment on them. Some offices or labs will require you to fill out and sign a consent form that gives permission to release the lab results to you.

Reading and understanding (interpreting) your blood test results.

All lab results have a column beside the title/name of the test that lists your "result" and there will also be a column that lists the "reference range" or "normal values" for each test. When you compare your result to the reference range, this will tell you where your result falls within the normal range. Most lab results that fall outside the normal values are "flagged" as abnormal or are highlighted.

The lab result page will either have an abnormal column for which to list the flagged results or they will have a notation beside the result such as "L" (meaning low) and "H" (meaning high).

Even results that are within the normal values are not always acceptable as being in a healthy range because with some tests, a borderline high or low level (on the edge of becoming abnormal) indicates the need for close observation and follow-up evaluations. Diseases, such as borderline diabetes and sub-clinical hormone deficiencies for example, are results that usually need to be followed up on (to monitor for development of full-blown disease).

Search the Internet to help you better understand your lab results.

If you do not understand what an abnormally high or low result on a particular test means, your doctor should help to inform you about them but you may also want to do a search on the Internet using the name of the blood test as the search term. You will find medical lab websites that will inform you as to what an abnormally high or abnormally low result means.

Thyroid Hormones and the Tests That Monitor Them

22

While some people may view this is a form of
self-treatment, this is not the case because doctors
are sometimes limited in their time for informing
patients thoroughly about their health disorders
and patients need a basic understanding of what
an abnormal result means for them. Gaining an
understanding of a health disorder versus
attempting to treat one, are not the same thing.
Doctors often have time limited to administering
treatment, without passing much information on
to the patient about their illness. It should be
recognized that patients have a right to know what
is affecting their lives and health. Simply gaining
some basic understanding about their illness will
not take away from the fact that they will still
need a licensed physician to treat them and to
prescribe the medications needed.

**If you feel you need a particular blood lab test
ordered, tell your doctor.**

This is another area that some people may see as
unnecessary patient involvement, however, being
proactive in your own lab testing and health care
through self-education and informed consultations
with your doctor can result in a higher quality of
care.

Thyroid Hormones and the Tests That Monitor Them

Doctors are not perfect and they cannot feel in your body what you do. They can treat you according to your symptoms but even this requires detailed input by the patient. If you have come across information online, through reputable medical sources that you feel is significant in regard to your case (i.e. blood tests needing ordered), you need to discuss this with your doctor.

I will admit, personally, that I have been to doctors who were opposed to any input from me as the patient and they were also opposed to my learning about my illness on fellow patient forums or reputable medical websites, while others have actually appreciated my pro-activeness because it helped them to better optimize my treatment.

The U.S. National Institutes of Health has a radio campaign that actually encourages patients to be more informative with their doctors and to ask them questions. The attitude of a doctor in this area may also help you decide whether he is the doctor for you or if you need to seek one who allows more cooperation from you.

Medical blood lab testing is the single most valuable diagnostic testing that is available. Without blood testing, many diseases and disorders, including thyroid hormone disorders would be much more difficult for medical professionals to diagnose.

Chapter Four

TSH for Monitoring Thyroid Hormone Therapy

While some of this information at the star of this chapter has already been covered in preceding chapters, some of the information bears repeating and additional perspectives regarding the TSH hormone will be added to the information that follows.

The, pituitary gland sends out the TSH hormone in varied amounts throughout the day to regulate the amount of thyroid hormones that are released from the thyroid gland.

When hypothyroidism develops, more TSH will be released from the pituitary gland, which sends a signal to the thyroid to produce and release more of its own hormones. If the pituitary senses that the thyroid is producing and sending out too much thyroid hormone into the body, it will then send less TSH to the thyroid. Less TSH is sent so that the thyroid is not being overly stimulated to continue providing the body with too much thyroid hormone, which is referred to as hyperthyroidism (overactive thyroid).

Thyroid Hormones and the Tests That Monitor Them

Since the discovery of TSH decades ago and how it can determine thyroid function through blood testing, it has become the single most commonly tested hormone level to monitor thyroid function. Not only is it used to detect an overactive or under-active thyroid gland, but it is also used to monitor patients who are being treated for either of these thyroid disorders to insure their treatments are getting proper results in correcting these two types of thyroid hormone imbalances.

In the year 2002, The American Association of Clinical Endocrinologists revised the normal range for TSH at blood testing labs to diagnose earlier cases of developing thyroid disorders. This revision was made due to the fact that these experts in the field of endocrine medicine believed that the previous TSH normal value range was too wide and would potentially miss many developing cases of thyroid hormone disorders.

The previous TSH range that blood testing labs were using was roughly "0.5 to 5.0 mIU/L" and the AACE recommended that the TSH normal values range be narrowed to "0.3 to 3.0".

This in their view will help to diagnose many more millions of patients with developing thyroid hormone imbalances, so that they can be recommended for follow-up testing or begin treatment earlier to prevent or slow down thyroid disease progression.

Statistics have revealed that thyroid diseases manifest more commonly in people who are between ages 35 and 40 and are at least five times more common in women than in men. Adults approaching their middle age years should have their TSH level tested as a precaution to detect possible developing thyroid disease, which increases in frequency among the elderly.

This again, is also more important for women, who more commonly develop thyroid hormone imbalances in their senior years. Younger women should also be tested during pregnancy, which also increases the risk for thyroid hormone imbalances.

Many new hypothyroid patients, who are started on thyroid hormone therapy, will have their treatment monitored by TSH testing only.

As we have learned, TSH is not a thyroid hormone but a pituitary gland hormone that reflects the T-4 and T-3 thyroid hormone levels. In most cases it does so accurately but in less common cases, TSH only testing can miss cases of inadequate treatment and cases of over-treatment as well.

This happens in patients whose TSH levels do not accurately reflect their thyroid hormone levels. While this is not common, it occurs often enough to demonstrate the need by treating doctors, to order tests of T-4 and T-3, along with TSH, for at least the first two or three blood retests to monitor thyroid hormone therapy.

Sometimes there is no clear explanation as to why TSH does not accurately reflect thyroid hormone levels in some patients. I have seen the testimonials of patients who had thyroid hormone levels that were at hypothyroid level but their TSH was in the normal range. When their pituitary function was also tested, to see if that was the problem, test results indicated normal pituitary function.

In these cases, there was no explanation for why TSH and the thyroid hormones were not correlating as they should (idiopathic – no explanation) but it is possible that the abnormal pituitary function was sub-clinical (mild hypopituitarism) but did not show up on pituitary function tests, as an overt problem. It could also be that the patient had other hormone imbalances such as adrenal or sex hormones, affecting the endocrine system as a whole (all hormone-producing glands) and causing a problem in communication between the pituitary and thyroid gland.

Giving myself as an example, I have an overall subtle endocrine dysfunction that causes me to need a very, suppressed TSH level, in order for my thyroid hormone therapy for hypothyroidism, to be effective. Unless my TSH is suppressed below normal, my thyroid hormone levels will not reach mid-range or above. While cases like mine are not common, they do exist and I have corresponded with other patients who experience this same scenario. If a doctor started out, testing only my TSH to monitor my thyroid hormone therapy, I would have been under-treated to this day.

Thyroid Hormones and the Tests That Monitor Them

While I'm not a doctor but rather a well-studied Thyroid Patient Advocate, I have corresponded with 100s of patients over the past several years and I have seen obvious patterns and have formed some strong opinions in regard to hypothyroid treatment and the blood retest monitoring of it.

Chapter Five

Newly Diagnosed/Treated Patients

If your doctor gives you a diagnosis of sub-clinical hypothyroidism and if it is the autoimmune type (Hashimoto's thyroiditis), as most hypothyroidism is in industrialized countries, a sub-clinical result on thyroid function tests, does not always tell you how severe the disease process is that is going on in your thyroid gland.

"Thyroid Autoimmunity" means your thyroid is being attacked by antibodies sent from your immune system that recognize your normal thyroid tissue, as a foreign invader, such as a virus, allergen or bacteria. This autoimmune process damages the thyroid gland and also causes it inflammation.The antibodies can also serve to block some of the thyroid hormone, so that it doesn't do the job it needs to, even when there is near-ample thyroid hormone available in your body. The fact is that patients have varying symptoms at the early stage of autoimmune hypothyroidism, caused by "Hashimoto's thyroiditis".

Thyroid Hormones and the Tests That Monitor Them

I also feel that newly treated hypothyroid patients need to be tested for TSH, Free T-4 and Free T-3, for at least the first couple of blood test repeats/follow-ups to monitor their thyroid hormone replacement therapy as previously mentioned. I mention this again because there are some patients whose TSH levels are not accurate in reflecting their thyroid hormone levels. Some patients must have their TSH suppressed very low before their thyroid hormone levels from the replacement therapy place their T-4 and T-3 at adequate levels for them (above mid-range and higher-normal).

As I also mentioned previously, I'm an example of a patient whose TSH needs suppressed more than the average patient. My average TSH blood retest result is at 0.005 which for the average patient, would be at seriously hyperthyroid level (over-treatment) but this only places my Free T-4 at mid-range and my Free T-3 at between mid-range and high-normal, where mine needs to be to provide me the needed symptom relief. My doctor knows for a fact that my TSH level does not accurately reflect my thyroid hormone levels.

On the other hand, some patients need a TSH that seems a little high for a treatment level but they experience toxicity (thyroid med induced hyperthyroidism) if their TSH goes below a 2.0. It's difficult to know which patients may be in these uncommon situations, unless the Free T-4 and Free T-3 are tested along with the TSH level.

By testing the TSH and thyroid hormones together for the first couple of follow ups after beginning thyroid hormone therapy, it can also detect another uncommon condition also discussed previously called "impaired conversion".

In these cases, TSH may be well suppressed from an adequate T-4 level but the even more active T-3 hormone is remaining low, for several possible reasons, some of which were discussed under the "Reverse T-3" subheading in Chapter One.

These are the types of patients who need a combination T-4 and T-3 medication or who need T-3 added to the T-4 they are already taking but this can only be determined when the T-4 and T-3 tests are added to TSH testing.

The possibility of these type problems are why I feel more thorough lab evaluation is needed to monitor new patients on thyroid hormone therapy.

<u>Chapter Six</u>

Differences between Diagnostic and Treatment TSH

I have received a number of e-mails from hypothyroid patients responding to articles I have written on the subject of "TSH testing". They are complaining of not feeling well, in spite of being on thyroid hormone replacement therapy and have included their most recent, follow-up lab results in their e-mails to me. In almost every one of these, their TSH levels are in the "normal" range for diagnosing hypothyroidism but they are not in the normal range for treating hypothyroidism and incredibly, they are stating in these e-mails that their doctors are saying that there is no difference between the two. There is however a difference between the two and we only need to look at reliable medical sources to know this and hopefully more thyroid treating doctors will be updated in regard to these facts.

The "diagnostic" TSH level, as revised by the AACE (American Association of Endocrinologists), in 2002, is roughly 0.3 to 3.0, as stated earlier.

Thyroid Hormones and the Tests That Monitor Them

The "treatment" TSH level they and other reputable medical sources recommend, is 1.0 to 2.0 for titrating (adjusting thyroid medication levels). Many patients feel better, at the 1.0 and even down to the lowest TSH normal level of just above 0.3.

Unfortunately, if a doctor uses the diagnostic TSH range, a patient may be receiving inadequate treatment because this would mean that they would recognize even the highest-normal TSH, as being sufficient treatment, when it often is not. For example, if a patient is treated on thyroid hormone replacement medication and their dose only suppresses their TSH down to 3.0, the doctor who is not using the treatment TSH targeted range, will recognize this level as being sufficient and the patient may continue to experience hypothyroid symptoms.

This scenario is made even worse, when the lab a doctor is using, is still using the old "diagnostic" TSH level of 0.5 to 5.0 that was revised by the AACE, to help diagnose cases of developing hypothyroidism earlier.

During my first two years of treatment for hypothyroidism, my first doctor kept my TSH between 3.01 and 4.95 and stated that even that higher level was "perfect". Well, it was not only inadequate thyroid hormone dosing, but I was virtually spinning-my-wheels and not getting very far with resolving my symptoms. Once finding a better informed doctor, who placed me on a combination T-4/T-3 replacement therapy and dosed me, to reduce my TSH level down to between 0.5 and 1.0, I felt better than I had in the three years previous. Afterward, through repeat blood retests, my doctor saw the need to suppress my TSH level even further, due to my TSH not being as accurate as it should be in reflecting my T-4 and T-3 thyroid hormone levels.

This Endocrinologist, who treats me now, agrees with many other Endo-doctors and thyroid specialists who will treat patients, getting their TSH levels down to lowest normal. A Thyroid Forum I used to post on frequently, that has a Board Certified Endocrinologist answering questions, repeatedly confirmed that his patients felt better with a TSH around 1.0 and that many of them he would replace with doses that would get their TSH down to between 0.5 and 1.0.

Thyroid Hormones and the Tests That Monitor Them

I believe patients should obtain copies of their most recent lab tests that were done in follow-up on their thyroid hormone therapy. The U.S. HIPAA Law entitles patients to copies of their medical lab tests results as previously mentioned. They should see if their TSH has been suppressed down closer to a 1.0 target range and if it hasn't been, they should discuss with their Doctor, using this as the target TSH level, to see if it better resolves their symptoms.

To repeat - the TSH that is used to diagnose thyroid disease, should not be the range used for treating hypothyroidism and both patients and doctors should be aware of this fact.

Some years ago, I found suggestions by some sources that comment on thyroid hormone therapy, in regard to suppressing TSH, which elevates with hypothyroidism, to almost undetectable levels before some patients experience symptomatic relief. I am now ashamed to admit it but this led me to finally experiment in this area, with my own medication, which I strongly and emphatically DISCOURAGE anyone from doing.

I did-so because of desperation for symptom relief from ongoing joint pain flare ups and severe fatigue spells I was experiencing at the time. I was involved in contract work requiring a lot of physical stamina and I needed a certain amount of wellness, to keep going. I very slowly increased my thyroid hormone medication, above that recommended by my Dr., until my TSH was almost undetectable.

I did not have any hyper/toxicity symptoms but experienced a severe, bone numbing fatigue, which means I likely was at the edge of dangerous reactions to the dose. My symptoms did not improve. I am now at the dose-level originally recommended by my doctor.

My opinion is that "certain" people have a pituitary response (gland that sends out TSH in response to thyroid hormone levels) that is sluggish but not actually at the "hypopituitarism" level (true hypo-functioning of the pituitary gland). Their Free T-3 and other levels can be upper, but not top-normal and their TSH will already be suppressed to near undetectable level. The problem is - how can a Dr. assume someone is in this category, when the majority of people are not?

Thyroid Hormones and the Tests That Monitor Them

This is why a standard is set that covers the majority of people treated for hypothyroidism. Most Endocrinologists and thyroid specialists, even the AACE (American Association of Clinical Endocrinologists), recommends a treatment TSH level below 3.0, so the goal of 0.5 to 1.0, is even more optimal. To narrow it even further, is simply too risky for the majority of people.

Hyper-toxicity (thyrotoxicity) from over-treatment (hyperthyroidism induced by too high a dose) can actually be life-threatening, due to possible development of serious heart arrhythmias and no-one should want to see that risk taken on wide scales but only with those individuals who apparently have the slight pituitary abnormality and need a little more attention in their unique cases. These people also need repeat blood retesting of their other thyroid hormone levels besides TSH (T4 and T3).

I think what happens is that someone who does obtain optimal symptom relief by symptomatic adjustment of their thyroid hormone dose, rather than by using the in-range cautions, believes their experience proves this success goes for everyone who might attempt this.

They are understandably very excited about it but in reality, the majority of people need a TSH level at the low-normal cut-off range but not below normal or they can be at serious risk for things like heart problems, hypertension and chronic bone loss (osteoporosis).

<u>Chapter Seven</u>

Thyroid Supplements Vs Thyroid Hormones

Recently, a lady e-mailed me, asking about certain over-the-counter supplements that are advertised to help optimize a person's thyroid function. She was struggling, as many patients do, with the idea of having to take a lifelong thyroid hormone replacement treatment. She was looking at the possibility of other options for treating her hypothyroidism. In this chapter, I am including my response to her on this subject, following below. Before I post that response I made to her, I would like to point out some important facts. While I believe there are natural supplements that will definitely improve a person's thyroid function, I do not believe these supplements can replace thyroid hormone replacement medications, needed by patients with advanced thyroid disease that has already caused hypothyroidism. It is my opinion, and one that I know agrees with that of medical professionals, that trying to replace thyroid hormone medication with a supplement containing no thyroid hormone, or an inconsistent amount, could actually be dangerous.

Thyroid Hormones and the Tests That Monitor Them

Hypothyroidism that is allowed to progress, due to lack of treatment or inadequate treatment can cause serious health problems, including heart disease, coma and eventual death.

Lack of thyroid hormone in the body, must be replaced and we cannot depend upon a supplement instead, that is supposed to increase our own thyroid function, when the thyroid has lost ground that cannot be regained, once permanently damaged due to disease.

Following now, is my response to the patient, who asked about certain thyroid supplements and her request for information about the differences between synthetic and natural thyroid hormone replacement medications. Respectfully, I used the term "brand" in place of the actual names of the over-the-counter supplements she asked about.

My Response:

"The two supplements you are looking into, are not thyroid hormones, they are supplements that are supposed to help a person's own thyroid gland to work at optimal level.

Thyroid Hormones and the Tests That Monitor Them

The problem is that a person with a diseased thyroid from Hashimoto's thyroiditis for example, cannot jump-start their thyroid past a certain point because once it is under-functioning, due to damage from auto-antibodies attacking it, regaining function of the gland cannot occur, no matter what is done, short of divine intervention.

That's not to say that some supplements would not still help to a certain degree because safe, helpful supplements being put into your body from the outside will have some effect (Some patients may take some of these in addition to thyroid medication if compatible).

The "brand #1 you asked about", is designed to stimulate your own thyroid but contains no actual thyroid hormones. It is advertised to "assist" in thyroid treatment, which means it is not a treatment itself but a supplement to treatment. The "brand #2 you asked about" is a bovine (beef) thyroid glandular, with the "thyroxin" taken out of it (extracted). This means they have to extract the thyroid hormone out of it, in order to sell it over-the-counter legally.

It is extremely difficult to get a supplement approved for non-prescription sales if it contains actual thyroid hormone. As far as the supplements go, you have to be careful to read the ingredients because Endocrinologists often warn patients that these "thyroid supplements" that contain no hormone, will not treat hypothyroidism and some contain ingredients that may actually work against thyroid medications.

With the fact of autoimmune thyroid disease not being able to be reversed, except in very rare cases, this would mean that even if those supplements worked to help strengthen the thyroid gland, how long would this improvement last? If the thyroid starts going downhill again once these supplements were stopped, this would mean they would have to be lifelong treatment as well. If auto-antibodies continued to attack the thyroid while on these non-hormone supplements, the gland would still eventually become so damaged over time, that there is no way they could continue to restore its function beyond a certain point and likely to no degree at all."

(End of Response)

To add a few more thoughts following my preceding response made to the woman inquiring my opinion in regard to thyroid boost supplements, I want to also mention that there are companies who market non-prescription natural "thyroid supplements", like those previously described but they know many doctors will not approve these in combination with thyroid hormone replacement.

In their attempt to bypass this problem, they will sometimes claim that you should take their supplement instead of a prescribed treatment for hypothyroidism.

It is possible that these type supplements would help boost a low functioning thyroid gland for a period of time but to claim they will reverse autoimmune thyroid disease is a false claim. If there were supplements that could do this, medical research would have discovered them many years ago.

Bottom line: Hypothyroidism must be treated with thyroid hormone replacement therapy and there is no alternative!

Thyroid Hormones and the Tests That Monitor Them

Are There Side-Effects Adjusting to a New Thyroid Hormone Dose?

Thyroid hormone replacement takes about eight weeks for a new dose to fully adjust within the body and to begin doing its job properly. Treatment can take longer however, depending on how many dose-adjustments are needed to get a patient to adequate/optimal levels. Many patients need one or two adjustments because Dr.s often start at a low dose and increase it upward which is called "titrating the dose". A patient should see more symptom-resolution as more weeks go by.

All types/brands of prescribed thyroid hormone are designed to take over the thyroid gland production of hormones, which is inadequate when hypothyroidism is present. As the hormone comes in from outside of the body, the pituitary gland (in the brain) senses the increase in the blood stream and sends less TSH to the thyroid gland (Thyroid Stimulating Hormone). For some hypothyroid patients, they will experience a break-even point, before improvement from increasing thyroid hormone levels begins to occur.

Chapter Eight

T-4 versus Combination T-4 and T-3 Hormone Medication

I will begin this chapter with three examples of thyroid hormone medications that are commonly prescribed in their brand name and generic forms.

The "Armour Thyroid" natural brand of thyroid hormone replacement medication contains a set dose of hormone, just like synthetic brands do. It is a combination T-4 and T-3 medication and contains 38mcg of T-4 (levothyroxin) 9mcg of T-3 (liothyronine) per each grain tablet (60mg).

The "Synthroid" brand is a T-4 only dose that comes in a variety of strengths from 25 to 300 mcg.

The "Thyrolar" brand is also synthetic but contains both T-4 and T-3 and is available in doses from 3.1 to 37.5mcg.

The only change a combination T-4/T-3 medication makes once it enters the body, whether it is a synthetic or natural brand, is that the T-4 in it, will partially convert into more T-3, if the body determines it requires more. The other possible change in the effectiveness of a dose would be the percent of absorption of it that can be affected by other things you are consuming at the time of taking your dose.

Taking calcium or iron, within 6-hours of taking thyroid medication (either type), can limit its absorption and the same is true of too much dietary fiber eaten too-close to thyroid hormone dosing, so these need to be consumed at least 6 hours apart from taking the daily dose.

I mention these things because there is misinformation out there in regard to the Armour Thyroid brand and other T-4/T-3 combinations that they are not consistent in pill-to-pill doses (that each same-strength tablet varies in strength). Forest Pharmaceuticals, the manufacturer of Amour, has been cleared by the FDA after finding them to not having dosage inconsistencies.

Synthroid, the major T-4 only brand of thyroid hormone medication recently went through the same approval in regard to dose consistency. The accusations that sometime arise against the hormone manufacturers are likely from Pharmaceutical wars for market shares, more than anything else.

I am not recommending Armour Thyroid brand over Synthroid as some advocates do because I believe some patients do better on Synthroid however I also believe the Armour brand is given an undeserved "bad rap", by Doctors who are simply parroting what the Pharmaceutical companies are telling them. The fact is that Synthroid has had bad press on it, just as Armour has. I maintain my own belief that patients need trial regimens of the opposite type medication, if they are tried on one brand and are not having success with it.

Is there a Need for Synthetic and Natural Thyroid Hormone?

I've read articles in regard-to how, in the early days of treating hypothyroid patients, they fed them raw animal thyroid glands.

The patients usually did very well on this strange method of treatment. Just the fact that thyrotoxicity (treatment-induced hyperthyroidism) happens with taking too high a dose of thyroid hormone replacement (patients attest to this happening today), is why safeguards are in place.

Is the system perfect? As you and I know, of course not. When patients don't respond favorably to the standard treatment, doctors need to look at every single area of the replacement to see if it can be tweaked (adjusted for improvement) even more. If every avenue has been explored in improving a patient's treatment, including exceeding the optimal dose (as agreed on between Dr. and patient), only then, should other causes for unresolved hypothyroid symptoms be looked into.

I am one of those patients who didn't do well on Synthroid, synthetic T-4 only medication and was switched to Armour brand – natural T4 and T3 combination and began doing much better. My mother however has been on Synthroid for many years and has done very well since being on it, with no need for switching her brand.

When I mentioned Armour to her several times in years past, asking if she thought she might do even better, she refused to inquire with her doctor about it because of feeling so well on the Synthroid and she didn't want to upset the applecart so-to-speak (why try fixing something that's not broken?).

I have read that some people actually have the opposite effect happen to them - they have bad reaction to Armour and are switched back to a synthetic brand (either T4 only or a combo T3 and T4). Some people for example, are allergic to porcine products, pork etc.... If Armour (made from pig thyroid glands) was the only brand available, what would happen to these hypothyroid people needing treatment?

Is Armour superior in treating hypothyroidism? For some people it absolutely is superior and extremely-so, in some cases. This may possibly be true in a majority of cases but synthetic still needs to be available for people who need another option, including those who cannot take the brand due to their religious affiliation, requiring kosher observance (consuming no pig by-products).

A patient's excitement and pro-activeness in advocating for a particular thyroid hormone brand, can be a good thing if done in the proper perspective and not taken to overboard levels. If enough treated hypothyroid patients begin to become proactive, this may someday contribute to causing reform of those things in regard to hypothyroid treatments that aren't good (i.e. treating according to lab ranges only, with no consideration for unresolved symptoms). This is true of those who advocate for the benefits of synthetic brands as well.

Thyroid Hormone Treatment Inadequacies

As far as the hormones taking over for the thyroid gland, so that it atrophies (stops working), this is actually the whole point of thyroid hormone replacement therapy. If a person waits until the thyroid gland completely stops functioning before starting thyroid medication, they risk death by myxedema coma. This is the dilemma, even for Doctors, to know at what point to actually start patients on hormone replacement, who are suffering only mild vases of hypothyroidism because it always results in the eventual shut down of the patient's own thyroid gland.

Symptoms are one of the most important reasons medication needs to be started but also, to reduce auto-antibody levels (a process that sometimes takes years) and to prevent goiter and nodules from developing (thyroid gland swelling and tumorous growths within it). From these facts, we can see that there are multiple reasons for starting replacement hormone medication in patients with developing hypothyroidism.

Many medical sources state that thyroid hormone medications also help to reduce thyroid auto-antibodies over time. Others believe it does not help reduce them and that natural brands of hormone may actually increase antibody levels. If antibody levels increase despite being on medication, this does not necessarily mean the medication is the cause but could be related to thyroiditis flares that happen commonly in chronic autoimmune hypothyroid disease patients.

There is an article published by The Journal of Clinical Endocrinology & Metabolism, titled: "In Search of the Impossible Dream? Thyroid Hormone Replacement Therapy That Treats All Symptoms in All Hypothyroid Patients".

The article points out the fact that many patients who are on hormone replacement therapy for hypothyroidism, do not always experience significant symptom relief.

The research study points out a variety of reasons for this problem of unsatisfactory results from thyroid hormone replacement designed to treat hypothyroidism.

It also points out the fact that some patients are treated with T-4 only thyroid medications, when some might benefit more from a combination T-4 and T-3 medication. It makes mention of the fact as well, that some patients may be under treated by their doctors with hypothyroid therapy in general.

While it is a very interesting study, I feel some mention of the fact that if hypothyroidism has "thyroid autoimmunity" as its cause, the disease itself has potential to cause symptoms apart from corrected thyroid hormone levels. There are many medical research studies in regard to this fact as well.

If thorough blood retesting is done to monitor hypothyroid therapy and levels are shown to all be adequate or even best-optimized and a patient is still experiencing unrelieved symptoms, other blood tests may need to be ordered, to rule out other possible causes for the unresolved symptoms. Thyroid patients are at higher risk for developing co morbid health disorders and these can potentially be mistaken for unresolved hypothyroid symptoms.

Chapter Nine

Symptoms of Thyroid Hormone Imbalance

It's always disappointing, hearing about a Dr. that won't treat a patient who has severe symptoms of under active thyroid, because their lab ranges aren't out of range enough yet. Thyroid hormone "receptors" can be blocked by the antibodies in cases of thyroid autoimmunity, causing hypothyroid symptoms, even with hormone levels in normal range, according to some medical sources.

Also, the antibodies can cause development of goiter and/or thyroid nodules (usually benign) as previously mentioned and thyroid hormone replacement medication can halt this or reduce already existing problems within the gland.

Some Dr.s who treat hypothyroidism are "lab-range only" ones and others look at these other issues listed above and other types of symptom-manifestations to determine the timing of starting a patient on treatment.

Some Dr.s claim it is their concern over making a patient go hyperthyroid (dose-induced thyrotoxicity) if they treat too early and that this can cause the previously-mentioned conditions of osteoporosis and heart arrhythmias however, the question would arise as to why can't they reassure against this through follow-up blood testing, just as they do with other patients on treatment for hypothyroidism? Medical websites I've researched claim that the osteoporosis possibility has been completely blown out of proportion and does not occur easily, unless a patient is severely over treated for long periods of time. As far as heart arrhythmias go, if they begin to occur (tachycardia – rapid heartbeat is common with over-treatment), a Dr. might simply reduce the dosage slightly, to alleviate this problem.

A patient should consider a second opinion if a doctor is reluctant to treat mild but symptomatic hypothyroidism but should be sure to take all lab results with them to a new doctor and always get copies of all labs each time tests are completed.

Some patients who become frustrated with not getting proper treatment will resort to self-treating with supplements or "thyroid booster" type herbals.

I personally would never use herbal methods to treat a thyroid disorder. I believe people who do, are playing with fire! You need Dr. Supervision and blood testing follow-ups for hypothyroidism to be treated properly.

I get very passionate about inadequate Dr. treatment of hypothyroidism but I have every confidence in the good ones who are out there doing a great job with their patients, of which there are many. There are plenty of good, quality physicians available to treat thyroid conditions but the trick is in finding them.

In regard to the antibodies involved in causing thyroid disease, there is no cure for them and they cause disease processes that are most often life-long. They do have to run their course, until a cure for thyroid autoimmunity is found but thyroid hormone replacement medication may significantly lower antibodies levels over time in some patients.

This demonstrates another positive reason for starting thyroid replacement medication in patients with the autoimmune type of hypothyroidism.

The antibodies will keep attacking until there's no more living thyroid tissue left to attack and so a patient who is not yet at a level of hypothyroidism that requires treatment, will reach that level at some point – some sooner than others.

Hypothyroid symptoms may include the following:

- constipation
- depression
- fatigue
- excessive need for sleep
- dry skin
- joint and muscle aches

Do Hyperthyroid Symptoms occur from Hypothyroid Therapy?

ALL thyroid medications have the same potential to cause heart arrhythmias and it is usually a matter of taking too much of any of them, that can cause this (the same warning on all prescribed-types applies). I take Armour brand T3/T4 replacement hormone but I was first was placed on too-high a dose of Synthroid T4-only, synthetic brand.

I didn't have any resulting heart arrhythmias but I did have other HYPER-thyroid type symptoms when I first started the over-treatment with Synthroid. When I was switched to Armour, I never once had these symptoms, due to my being placed on a lower starting dose, that was slowly titrated upward to an optimal level.

For some patients, the opposite occurs and they experience hyperthyroid symptoms when taking hormone brands, like Armour that contain T3 in them, regardless of whether their dose is administered at proper levels, because of their sensitivity to it.

I've read online testimonials by people who are more sensitive to the Armour brand (natural T4/T3) than to the Synthroid (synthetic T4). I believe this is because Armour (made from pig/porcine thyroid glands) has both hormones in it and medical researchers say T3 has more potential to cause hyper type symptoms such as arrhythmias than the "T4 only" medications do.

This does not mean that Armour is not superior in the long-term for these patients, if they are given time to adjust to the medication properly.

A patient can also naturally go from hypo to hyper thyroid with autoimmune thyroiditis and many patients attest to this as well (i.e. spells of Hashitoxicosis or flares of thyroiditis). I too, early-on with my Hashimoto's, had severe anxiety and was frequently awaking during the night in cold sweats etc..., while I also experienced short-term but rapid weight-loss. Mine finally went from this temporary state of hyperthyroid symptoms, to progressive hypothyroidism and it has stayed there but occasionally I do have some anxiety symptoms that I believe to be caused by fluctuations in either my thyroid hormone levels or changes in the thyroid antibodies levels (possibly both are involved).

Medical websites I've researched say that both hypo and hyper thyroid patients can experience anxiety symptoms as a manifestation of thyroid autoimmunity, regardless of corrected hormone levels and that this can be the case even when the hypothyroidism is at a subclinical level. In regard to the hyperthyroid swings, that then go back to hypothyroid phases in Hashimoto's patients, this is reported by medical sources, to be due to the antibodies attack against the thyroid gland as I have described.

The response by the thyroid gland, while it is still able, is to release large spurts of hormone in attempt to compensate against damage that is being done to it by the autoimmunity. We, in a sense have germ warfare going on in our bodies you might say! You'll see mentioned on some medical sources the fact that Hashimoto's thyroiditis patients commonly have hyperthyroid swings until the gland becomes so damaged that it can no longer fight back against the immune system attacking it with these mysterious auto-antibodies (it remains a mystery as to why our own immune systems can begin to attack us).

Hyperthyroid symptoms from any cause (i.e. Graves' disease, thyroid nodules or over-treated hypothyroidism) may include the following:

• rapid heart rate
• diarrhea
• anxiety and nervousness
• sweating
• tremors
• insomnia
• muscle weakness

See a qualified medical doctor if you believe you may be experiencing symptoms indicating the need to be tested for abnormal thyroid hormone levels. An early diagnosis can help to prevent a worsening of symptoms, that can in some cases take a considerable amount of time for patients to see full recovery from. This would include myxedema (body tissue swelling), thyroid eye disease and co-morbid nutritional deficiencies.

It is my hope that the chapters of this book have helped readers to better-understand the function of thyroid hormones and how blood-tested levels of them can detect developing diseases of both the hyperthyroid and hypothyroid types.

(END)